Yoga

INDIA IN A NUTSHELL (BOOK 1)

OBAIDUR RAHAMAN

Copyright © 2018 Obaidur Rahaman

All rights reserved.

No part of this book may be reproduced in any form by any electronic, mechanical, photocopying, recording, or any other means without permission in writing from both the copyright owner and the publisher.

ISBN: 1981455523
ISBN-13: 978-1981455522

To Swami Vivekananda

CONTENTS

What the hell is water? 1
What is not yoga? 3
Reading the book of life...5
What is yoga? 7
Yoga and liberation..9
The side effects of yoga 12
How to do yoga?...15
Raja yoga or the path of meditation 17
Karma yoga or the path of action..................................19
Jnana yoga or the path of knowledge 22
Bhakti yoga or the path of devotion...............................24
What now? 26
Afterword 28

ACKNOWLEDGMENTS

I am grateful to everyone who helped me writing this book:

Sarah Barakah for editing the manuscript, for the feedback on the cover design and for being an invaluable part of the journey to explore this ancient practice together and to share it with people,

Yoko for the beautiful cover design,

Dalia Ibrahim for feedback on the cover design,

the beautiful people in Weimar who gave me a chance to teach them yoga,

Culture Talk at the Bauhaus Universität Weimar for inviting me to give a presentation on yoga which has helped me to write the first draft of the manuscript.

OBAIDUR RAHAMAN

What the hell is water?

"There are these two young fish swimming along, and they happen to meet an older fish swimming the other way, who nods at them and says, 'Morning, boys, how's the water?' And the two young fish swim on for a bit, and then eventually one of them looks over at the other and goes, 'What the hell is water?'"
~*David Foster Wallace.*
Think about this story for a little bit.

What is this story about? I want you to take a couple of minutes to really think about it before you read on.

So, what do you think it is about? I don't know about you but when I heard this story for the first time I was terribly disturbed. Its implication is heart wrenching.

Are we all not like that fish? Not the old one, but the young one? The fish was born in the water and lived in it ever since. He is surrounded by water all the time, almost every moment of his life. And yet, he does not know what water is.

Why? Because he is so used to it that he does not think about it anymore. He does not feel it. He does not notice it.

The situation is the same with most of us. We are all submerged in this mysterious world around us and yet we go on living without noticing it.

When we were little children, we knew how exciting it was. If you watch little children you will see how curious and joyous they are about everything. Be it the simplest of things, like a puddle of water or a colorful insect or a piece of rock - everything is interesting and enjoyable.

But now we are so preoccupied with the problems of life and the daily routine that we don't feel what it really means to be alive anymore.

We got used to living. So much so that we don't feel alive anymore. Except for a few special moments when something touches our souls deeply, we are vegetating, not living.

And then some of us get in the trap of setting high goals to give a meaning to our lives. Chasing a dream. Trying to live in the future. If we fail to reach the goal it brings frustration. If we succeed, it brings disillusionment. Because other than momentary satisfaction it does not bring any happiness.

It seems that we are all doomed to suffer like this. But is there no way out of it?

It turns out that there are ways, and yoga is one of them.

What is not yoga?

There are a number of misconceptions about what yoga really is and why one should do yoga. Unfortunately, this number is increasing at an alarming rate.

When I ask these questions to people, I get typical answers like these:

-Yoga is a type of fitness exercise.

-It helps you to lose weight.

-It makes you flexible, fit, healthy and strong.

-It connects your body and mind.

-It helps you to realize inner peace and well-being.

These are the answers given by people who have done some kind of yoga at least once in their lives.

There are also people who have never done yoga. Most of them believe that if you can stay at some impossible body posture or stand on your head or something like that, you are in yoga.

And there are also the intellectual/scientist types. A smart-looking guy once told me,

"These days I see all these people doing yoga. It is considered as something so cool and hip. If you are not doing it, you are uncool."

"It is true, indeed. But have you ever tried it?"

"No, I normally stay away from silly trends."

Another time I overheard a young man saying this to his friend,

"Oh, you are a scientist, of course you don't believe in yoga."

I was speechless.

It is essential to understand what yoga is in order to benefit from it. First, let's try to understand what yoga is not.

The physical aspect of yoga is only a tiny part of it. There is a name for the body postures that people take for yoga. It is called asana. Asana is a very small part of yoga. Asana is not yoga.

Asana can help you to live a long healthy life. But if you only care for your body, a healthy body is the only thing you will get. But is there something more to care for?

To practice yoga, there is nothing one needs to believe in. You should never believe in something without evidence or experience. Yoga is not a faith.

Reading the book of life

We cannot fully appreciate the value of something when we get it without working for it. For example, our own lives.

We are born as humans but we played no role in it. Consequently we neither understand nor appreciate life. We don't appreciate the miracle of being a human, being able to feel, being able to think, being able to take actions.

When we were born, we did not know how our bodies functioned, how our minds worked, what we were capable of doing. We were utterly helpless. We constantly needed our parents to survive.

As we grew, we learned how to survive in this crazy world. Most of us are still striving to gather all the necessities to live a comfortable life. Some of us reached that goal and stayed there. And a very few looked beyond.

Essentially, most of us explored ourselves as little as necessary to survive. The rest of that vast ocean of who we are, especially our inner world, is left unexplored.

What a pity.

You are like a book. The book contains all the knowledge of the universe. It is a book full of colors, pictures and amazing stories. The physical part of the book is your body and the knowledge inside it is your spirit.

Unfortunately you cannot read the book because it is written in a foreign language. Nevertheless you take good care of the book itself. Just like you put a nice cover on a book, keep it in a safe place and dust it regularly, you feed your body, you dress it, you decorate it, you do whatever it takes to keep it healthy and beautiful.

Occasionally you open the book, flip through the pictures and get a glimpse of the wonders hidden in it. These are the rare moments in your life when you get to know your innermost self and it touches you deeply.

But most of the time you are so caught up with the body that you do not have the time to look inside you.

It's a pity.

Yoga is a way to decipher the book of life. Yoga is a way to go beyond the body, into the inner self. Ironically most people think that yoga is nothing but a means for good health and relaxation.

Pity?

What is yoga?

The apparent difference between any two objects in the universe is only superficial. Deep down they are identical.

That means you and me, the towel and the trees, the moon and the monkey, all are exactly the same thing. The differences in the size, shape, color, location, etc. are nothing but illusions.

There is an agreement between science and religion about this fact. The big bang theory suggests that the whole universe came into existence from a point of infinite density, called singularity. Since everything in the universe came from this point, they are essentially the same.

Likewise all the religions of the world have been telling us for a long time that god is in everything. Everything is just an expression of the same thing.

For example, gold can be melted and given the

shape of a ring, a necklace or a bangle. Although these objects have different sizes and shapes, they are essentially made of the same thing, gold.

Science tells us that everything in this universe is made up by different forms of energy and types of elementary particles. These particles are in constant flux with their surroundings. The atoms that constitute my body today can be a part of the soil tomorrow and part of the tree the day after.

The singularity described by science can be understood intellectually. Likewise, the god proposed by religion can be believed as the truth.

But there is yet another way of knowing it other than by intellect or belief.

It can be experienced, directly.

A few thousand years ago, some people in what is called India today discovered something interesting. They discovered that by gradually concentrating the mind they could attain a supreme state of being. In that state they could experience themselves as identical to the rest of the universe. It was a state of ultimate liberation and complete self-knowledge. This experience has been described by many words like *nirvana, moksha, samadhi* or enlightenment.

Although possible, the attainment of *nirvana* was extremely difficult. So they developed a step-by-step method to realize it systematically. Although it is a long and arduous path, if followed persistently, it can be realized.

This path toward *nirvana* by increasing concentration and self-awareness is called yoga.

The word *yoga* itself means "union". Union of the body, mind, soul and the universe.

Yoga and liberation

Why should we do yoga? We should do yoga to realize *moksha* or liberation. We cannot experience ourselves as the universe without completely liberating ourselves.

But liberating from what? What is preventing us from being free? Let's try to understand that first.

Imagine you are walking on the street in the morning. Suddenly you see a man approaching you. That man insulted you last night in front of your friends. The moment you see his face, resentment and hatred rise in your mind. Subsequently you avoid him or behave in a hostile manner.

But why do you hate him today when he did not do anything bad to you today? You hate him today because he did something bad to you yesterday. Your action at the present moment is based on the memory of yesterday. Maybe you don't need to be hostile to him today, but you cannot help it.

Similarly you love somebody today based on past memories. If you think carefully, you would realize that almost everything you do is determined by the memory of your past experiences.

Now, there is nothing wrong with having memories. They prevent us from making the same mistakes again. They guide us to do things better today than yesterday.

But there is a downside to it.

The mind, which deals with the memory, has a small conscious part and a large and powerful unconscious part. Most of the time the conscious part is sleeping, and the unconscious part is deciding our actions based on the past memories.

What does it mean? It means that most of the time we are not conscious of ourselves. Reason, rationality and free will can function only when we are consciousness. But, in a way, most of the time we are asleep. Most of the time the unconscious mind is deciding our actions based on past memories, not on reason, which requires present moment awareness.

Now, if past memory is the only thing that decides our action at the present moment, we are completely on autopilot mode. This is similar to living the life of an animal.

Life can be summarized as cycles of memories and actions. Memories decide the actions and the actions create new memories. These cycles are also known as habits. We are slaves of these habits.

These cycles of memory and action exist because of a good reason. They are crucial for our survival. But they come with a cost. If you think a little bit, you will realize that many of the sufferings in our lives are directly related to it.

If you want to just survive, you are well equipped for it already. But if you want to liberate yourself from these vicious cycles, you have a tool at your disposal: Yoga.

The side effects of yoga

Ideally yoga should be practiced for the realization of *moksha* or liberation and not for benefits. A yogi would naturally enjoy the benefits as by-products.

Yoga is like a ripe mango. It has a colorful skin, texture and aroma. Most people are attracted by its external beauty. They understand yoga by the physical postures or the asanas. People who are only doing asanas are essentially licking the skin of the mango. They have little idea about the sweet, juicy nectar that is hidden inside.

So what are the benefits of yoga?

First we need to understand something important. The fact that we are capable of being conscious does not mean that we *are*. We are not always conscious. In fact, we rarely use this ability. Most of the time we are on autopilot mode.

Being conscious means being alive. If we are not

conscious, we are not living life in its full glory. Whichever simple thing we do, when we do it automatically or compulsively, we miss it altogether. It is as good as sleepwalking. But when we do it consciously, we feel it, we live it, we experience it with our innermost being. Yoga improves the quality of our lives by making us more conscious.

Most of the sufferings in our lives are caused by the inability to see things as they are. Our minds are so hopelessly polluted by the memories of our past experiences that we are unable to see things as they are. Yoga helps us to see everything more clearly.

Through the practice of yoga, we gain the ability to deal with our bodies, minds, thoughts and emotions. We gain calmness and peace.

Yoga sharpens our minds.

The execution of every task in our daily lives requires concentration of mind. But the mind is like a monkey, a monkey that got drunk and then bitten by a snake. We are inefficient in whatever we do because our minds never rest in one place.

For example, a needle can penetrate fairly tough material with a little force. The secret of its power is the accumulation of the force in its tip. The tip has a small surface area. The ability to penetrate is determined by the pressure, which is measured by the force divided by the surface area. So given a particular force, the smaller the surface area, the higher its ability to penetrate.

Similarly when our minds are focused, we get things done much faster and with better results. So if you think that you do not have the time to do yoga, you need to understand that yoga creates more free time than it consumes.

By regular practice of yoga you can gain tremendous reading speed, good memory and so on.

Yoga also brings flexibility, good health and well-being.

How to do yoga?

When we truly understand what yoga is and why one should do it, the how part becomes easier. Because the what part gives you clarity and the why part gives you motivation.

Yoga is a path, and there are more than one path.

The same way you can reach the central square of a city by following different streets, liberation can be realized by following different types of yoga. They all ultimately lead you to the same destination.

However, one needs to be careful.

Since yoga has become a fashionable thing, many people are exploiting it as an opportunity to make money. They have created a plethora of easy-to-follow, entertaining, sometimes superstitious, sometimes totally nonsensical, new-age methods. And these new forms of yoga are selling like hot cakes. If you fall for them, you will not only waste your time but also be mislead, lost, even harmed.

This is why it is important to understand which yoga is authentic and which is not.

The root of yoga can be traced back to different religions in ancient India. For example, Hinduism, Buddhism, Jainism, etc.

In fact, it goes beyond the origin of these religions. Thus, yoga can be practiced without the requirement of faith.

You are free to explore different types of yoga and use your own judgment to figure out which one is authentic and whether it appeals to you. Please take this as a guide and do some of your own research.

For now we will explore four major types of yoga originated in Hinduism:

1. Raja yoga or the path of meditation
2. Karma yoga or the path of action
3. Jnana yoga or the path of knowledge
4. Bhakti yoga or the path of devotion

Before we start exploring, please note that testing out all of these paths is generally a good idea. But continuously jumping from one to the other would prevent you from gaining any reasonable progress and benefit. Sticking to one path and going where it ultimately leads you is absolutely necessary.

But at the same time it is good to know that these paths are harmonious to each other. They will all help you to go forward.

Raja yoga or the path of meditation

Raja yoga is one of the mainstream paths of yoga. It has eight steps. The practice of a higher step is only possible if one meticulously follows the steps leading to it.

The eight steps are the following:

Yamas: If you practice yoga but do not live a life that goes along with it, you will have no progress. Your surroundings, your body, your mind and your life style constitute the foundation on which the practice of yoga is built. Therefore it is vital to live a life of non-violence, truthfulness, chastity, etc.

Niyamas: Discipline and structure are necessary to achieve anything significant. Yoga requires cleanliness of body, mind and speech. It also requires introspection, acceptance and persistence.

Asana: The ability to sit in a comfortable body posture or asana is a prerequisite for meditation.

Among all the asanas that help to keep the body strong and healthy, Padmasana or the lotus posture is very important because it is possible to sit in this posture for a long time. During mediation it is important to keep the spine, the neck and the head erect.

Pranayama: It is a set of techniques to consciously regulate breathing. The practice of pranayama gradually enhances the mind's ability to focus. This ability is then extended to regulate the nervous system, internal organs and flow of energy in the body.

Pratyahara: The mind continuously and compulsively generates thoughts, even when we are sleeping. The practice of pratyahara enables the mind to stay detached from both thoughts and the sensory world.

Dharana: Once the mind is able to remain detached for a while, it can be trained to focus on a single object. Dharana is the practice of holding the mind at one inner object for a time period, without any distraction.

Dhyana: You can think of dhyana as a deeper stage of dharana.

Samadhi: As the mind's ability to concentrate intensifies, there comes a state when the thinker, the thought and the object of thinking all become one.

Karma yoga or the path of action

This is an important path of yoga because we are doing actions all the time.

Actions are determined by a person's belief system. Crudely speaking, a good person does good things and a bad person does bad things.

This is obvious. What is not so obvious is that the actions can also alter the belief system.

Our belief systems and personalities can be changed by our actions as well. To put it simply, if somebody performs good actions over and over, the person becomes good.

This is why it is very important to do the right actions in the right ways. But what are the right actions and how can we do them? Karma yoga gives the answers.

What are the right actions?

Karma yoga says that the unselfish actions are the

right actions. Many of our sufferings are caused by the inability to see things as they are. This is mostly because of our self-centeredness and self-obsession, seeing ourselves as different from others. Selfless actions help us to see ourselves and the world as the same thing. They help us to dissolve our ego.

And what is the right way to do actions?

Since childhood, we are brainwashed to live goal-oriented lives. First we calculate the benefits, set goals and then take actions. There are millions of books, articles, websites, seminars, podcasts and videos that are luring us to fulfill our dreams by thinking big and setting high goals. This is complete insanity.

When we dream and obsess about goals we try to live in the future. But we are never successful because life is happening now, at this moment.

Karma yoga suggests we live exactly in the opposite manner.

There is a causal relationship between any action and its result. If we do good actions, good results will follow. If we do bad actions, bad results will be born from them. It is a universal rule. The mechanism of karma yoga is based on this rule.

Once we understand this, we do not need to worry about the result, but just need to make sure that the action is good and to do it with dedication. The worrying about the result reduces a person's ability to focus on the action and to enjoy it.

Also, always thinking about the benefit terribly restricts our actions. We want to undertake only those actions that might bring some benefits as portrayed by our limited imagination.

But the world is tremendously complex. There are

numerous factors continuously interplaying with each other. An action can bring a result that is completely unimaginable at the time of setting the goal.

Thus, we will deprive ourselves from some wonderful results if we neglect certain actions because of our inability to see the future.

We are unable to see the future, but we are able to choose the right actions.

Jnana yoga or the path of knowledge

Knowledge can also lead to *moksha*. This is the preferred path of the intellectuals.

However, as we have learned before, an intellectual understanding of the oneness of the self with the universe is not the same as *moksha*. It needs to be experienced.

Nonetheless, intellectual understanding can be a step toward *moksha*. For example, as a part of *jnana* yoga.

Yogis say that we fail to experience ourselves as identical with the universe because of *avidya* or ignorance.

What is this ignorance?

It is the ignorance about who we are. We usually identify ourselves as our bodies. But this is not accurate. This is not the complete picture of who we really are.

Yogis say that this ignorance can go away if one starts by asking the question "Who am I" and pursues it carefully to where it leads to.

The question "Who am I" leads to further questions like:

"Am I the body?"

"Am I the thoughts in my mind?"

Or "Am I the mind?"

A careful introspection confirms that I am none of these. Not even the mind. But I am the pure consciousness or awareness that is behind all these. The physical world is just an expression of it.

Although it appears like it, *Jnana* yoga is not a theory. It is a method that can be practiced.

The practice of *jnana* yoga consists of three steps:

Listening: Start by gaining the knowledge of the scriptures like Upanishads and Vedanta. Traditionally they were recited by the gurus and listened to by the disciples.

Thinking: Just learning the scriptures by heart is not enough. One needs to contemplate on them, understand them, ask questions and clarify all the doubts and confusions.

Meditating: When a clear grasp of the concepts is achieved, one needs to meditate on them. The meditation will ultimately lead to self-realization.

Bhakti yoga or the path of devotion

We all have emotions, in various forms and flavors. It could appear as love, it could appear as hatred, it could be stressful or pleasant.

Bhakti yoga works by giving a higher direction to these emotions. It is a path of loving devotion toward a supreme being. You can call that god or the universe. It is your choice.

Most religions in the world follow this path, in some forms or other.

Since it is difficult to offer devotion to the universe as a whole, certain symbols and images are used for worshipping. The early devotional practice typically involves worshipping a personal god, specific rituals and mythology. But it is important to understand that true bhakti yoga goes beyond them to the ultimate goal of liberation.

Since all religions eventually lead to the same goal, a

devotee should not hate or criticize other religions.

On the other hand one needs to sincerely follow one path and not continuously shift from one to the other. No real progress will come that way.

Although the path of devotion is easy and natural for human beings, numerous superstitions and horrific fanaticism rotate around its early forms. People take the superficial aspects of it too seriously and forget that it is just a tool to attain liberation.

Thus, bhakti yoga should be practiced carefully, always keeping its purpose in mind.

What now?

Have you got a question?

If you have a question, do not just go back to surfing the internet or checking messages on your phone and forget about the question.

If you have a question, seek the answer.

Seek the answer with sincerity, integrity and patience. We do not find the answers to many of our questions simply because we do not make the necessary effort.

Be a seeker. If it is an important question for you, seek the answer.

We just learned about what yoga really is and a few options of practicing it.

Most of us enjoy having options. You might want to follow a path of yoga that suits your personality or is easier for you to practice.

If you are an introvert, Raja yoga might be the right

path for you. If you are an intellectual, Jnana yoga might be the right path for you. If you are an active and energetic person, Karma yoga might be the right path for you. If you are an emotional person, Bhakti yoga might be the right path for you.

You will have to explore and find out. The sooner you find it the better. Because then you can start making some real progress. The following books are recommended for further reading:

Raja Yoga
Karma Yoga
Jnana Yoga
and
Bhakti yoga
by
Swami Vivekananda.

These four paths are not the only paths toward liberation. There are a few more genuine paths. If you prefer, you can follow one of them and it will ultimately lead you to the same destination.

However, it is important to understand the basic principles of the path and follow them with sincerity and compassion, both to yourself and to others. Be non violent and stay away from over emphasis on rituals and fanaticism.

And always use your own reason and judgment.

I wish you all the best in your spiritual journey. Namaste.

Afterword

I feel very lucky to be born and raised in the incredible land of India. From early on, I was exposed to the culture, arts and science that developed there since ancient times. I feel great pleasure to share some of these with you. This is the reason I started this series.

I hope you enjoyed reading this book. I need your help in order to make it available to as many people as possible.

You can help me by telling your family and friends about this book and by writing a favorable review of the book online.

Thank you very much for your valuable time and support!

Obaidur

About the Author

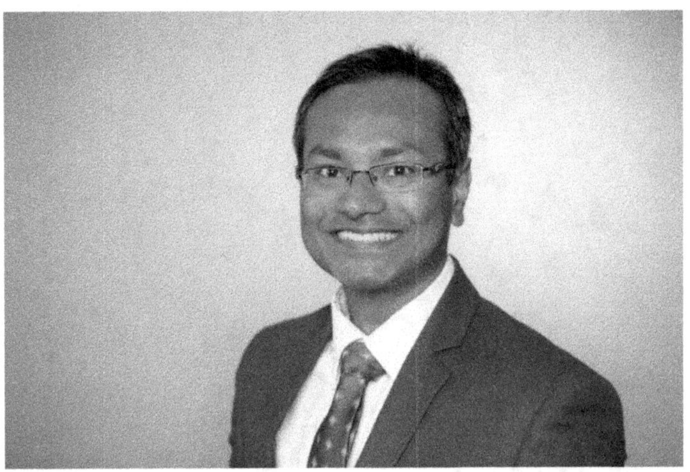

Dr. Obaidur Rahaman, a native of India and a graduate of Indian Institute of Technology Bombay, obtained his PhD degree in computational chemistry from University of Delaware, USA. Obaidur lives in Weimar, Germany with his wife and son. When he is not in his office staring at the molecule on the computer screen, you might find him in the beautiful Ilm Park staring at the trees or at the fish in the river.

To get updates about upcoming books you can visit Dr. Obaidur Rahaman's website here:

http://www.ObaidurRahaman.com/

www.ingramcontent.com/pod-product-compliance
Lightning Source LLC
Chambersburg PA
CBHW070751260726
48660CB00007B/3071